YOUR KNOWLEDGE HAS VALUE

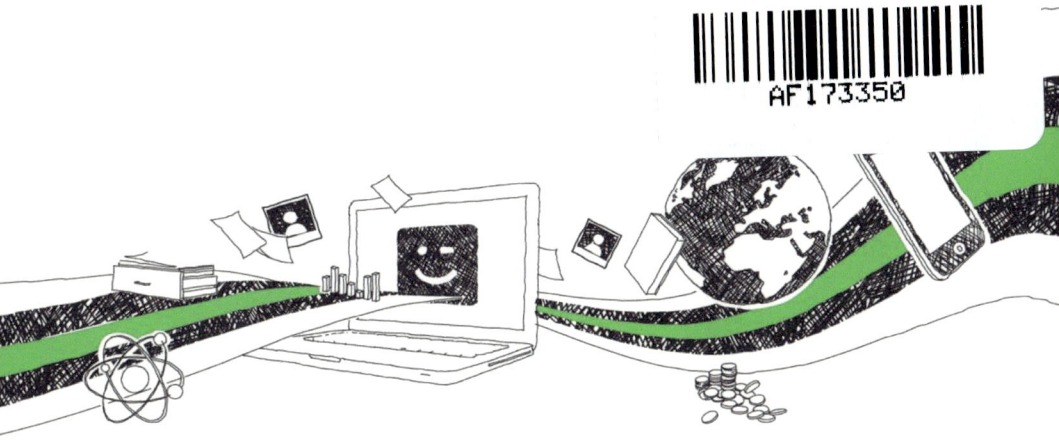
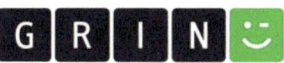

Susanne Obermaier

Comparison of the German and the British welfare system

GRIN Verlag

Bibliografische Information der Deutschen Nationalbibliothek:

Die Deutsche Bibliothek verzeichnet diese Publikation in der Deutschen National-
bibliografie; detaillierte bibliografische Daten sind im Internet über http://dnb.d-
nb.de/ abrufbar.

Imprint:

Copyright © 2009 GRIN Verlag GmbH
Druck und Bindung: Books on Demand GmbH, Norderstedt Germany
ISBN: 978-3-656-11311-9

This book at GRIN:

http://www.grin.com/en/e-book/187779/comparison-of-the-german-and-the-british-
welfare-system

Comparison of the German and the British welfare system

International comparison of welfare states

Nonprofit-, Social- & Healthcare Management 2007
WT 2009 / 2010

Table of Content

How are the German and the British social security systems comparable? What are the problems when evaluating welfare states?

1 Social security system – Germany

1.1 Historical background

Germany as well as Austria are pioneers on the field of social security provided by the state. The beginnings reach back to the 19th century – when following insurances were developed:

- 1883 health insurance
- 1884 accident insurance
- 1889 old-age insurance/diability insurance
- 1927 unemployment insurance
- 1995 the compulsory long term care insurance

The chancellor Bismarck wanted to prevent a revolution of the socio-democratical party so he developed the social insurance law. During the industrial revolution the economical and social problems got really critical (e.g. accident danger in fabrics). Still in the very beginning the social insurance was by far not enough to cover the basic needs of human. The fee and the performance are coherent because the insurance was established for the employees that basically excludes the thought of minimum collateral. Germany still is a "conservative welfare state" or in other words Germany owns the "Bismarck Model".
In the decades after world war II the insurance system extended and benefits and members enlarged.
In the 1950s the government decided to bind the insurance on the income of the people. In the 70s the German economy shrank because of the demographical change and rising unemployment rates and a lot of cut-backs had to take place. Also in the 90s when both parts of Germany reunited it was a big challenge for the social security system. But despite all prognosis it was quite a stable change.[1] The German system still seems to be quite stable but the annuity insurance is endangered for there are demographically too less people to carry the financial burden of the insurance.[2]

1.2 Political background

The federal constitution insists that Germany is a social federal constitution. Slogans like "freedom", "equality" and "solidarity" from the French revolution are part of the socio-ethical context in Germany. So there are rights and responsibilities for every

---

[1] Schmid 2002
[2] Seidl/Jickeli 2006

citizen.[3] There is also the principal of subsidiary which means the smaller unit has to be prioritized.[4] There are three more basic principles for the social security system:

- Insurance
- Care
- Provision
-

These three regulate the risk provision and the protection of the citizen from social emergencies and the way of payment.

The German social insurance insists that social risks are predictable as well as the coverage with fees. But still it is not individual but collective. The service is not strictly connected with the fee. The principle of provision includes compensation for special sacrifices for the state (e.g. post war injuries, appointee). The principle of care is based on the legal right for people living below the poverty limit to be provided with basics for everyday living.

The acceptance for the insurance system is the highest.[5]

1.3 Individual insurance

The German social insurance system is not only one of the oldest systems but also one of the most comprehensive. The coverage of the social service expanded constantly over the last decades since World War II.[6]

1.3.1 Pension system

The German pension system is based on the so called "generation contract". This means that the generation which is currently working pays the pension of the people who are in pension. The aim is to keep the life standards of people in pension, which means that the pension gets customized to the current salary and price development. The pension is equivalent to the wages earned in past times. The pension is mainly financed through fees. Each employer and employee pays half of the fee. The government pays grants for the not insured services. The amount of the pension is calculated on the basis of special formula.[7]

1.3.2 Health care

In 2002 there were 357 health insurance companies. There are regionally, sectorally and occuptationally structured. Every citizen is free to choose the insurance company and the companies are obliged to contract. Since 1994 there is a risk structure compensation payment. This compensation payment was established to balance salary of contribution of members, number of family member who are freely insured and age and sex of the insured people. This system makes all insurance companies

---

[3] Schmid 2002
[4] Blüm/Zacher 1989 as cited in Schmid 2002
[5] Schmid 2002
[6] Schmid 2002
[7] Schmid 2002

competitive. Generally there is the principle of solidarity. That means that the financial stronger person pays for the financially weaker person (e.g. elder people). In 2009 there was a great health care reform. One of the major changes is that the amount of the fee is not regulated by the companies itself but by the government. Employees pay 8,5 % of the wage and employer pay about 7,5% into the health care fund. Another change is that physicians will not be paid based on a bonus system but rather on a lump-sum payment. Especially this change causes a lot of resistance already. In Germany it is obliged to be insured. [8]

1.3.3 Family

Families with children get monthly support from the state depending on the amount of children. After the second child the support rises constantly. The support does not depend on the income of the parents.
Maternity leave is just like Work- and Health care prevention as well as child-raising allowance an important support of family policy. Maternity leave is for women being employed and includes job protection six weeks before and eight weeks after delivery. Maternity allowance does not depend on citizenship and family status. The allowance is as high as the clear salary of the last three month.[9]

1.3.4 Accident

The most important function of the accident insurance is prevention. Service of the insurance companies includes prevention of accidents and its risks through information and security instructions. But also services which keep the employee and his/her family from the consequence of working accidents or industrial disease are provided. In this case the insurance pays allowances, care and therapies. In these cases it does not matter by whom fault the accident happened. Even accidents on the way to the working place are covered by the insurance.[10]

1.3.5 Unemployment

The unemployment insurance has to be remunerated both from the employer and the employee. Age, family status affects the amount and length of how long the allowance will be provided.[11] In Germany as well as in GB only people who can not work will get welfare. Since 2005 there are three steps in the german system:
- the unemployment allowance (ALG)
- poverty proved allowance (ALHI)
- highly poverty proved allowance (SOHI)
-

---

[8] Braasch 2007
[9] Schmid 2002
[10] Schmid 2002
[11] Schmid 2002

Only when one overlaps these procedures one is allowed to get the allowances. The SOHI is the last social net for the citizen. For long-term unemployed Germany constructed a help system these citizen get ALG II.[12]

2 Great Britain

2.1 Historical background

1834 the first British social security net was established, the so called "Poor law". The reason to do so was the early industrialisation which made many people living under the poverty line. The needy citizen had to work in working houses and do the jobs they were able to do. In the 19th century other forms of social security developed. "Friendly societies", insurance companies and trade unions were established to keep citizens from poverty caused by age or illness. 1911 the social insurance was developed. The 1897 developed "workmen compensation act" already lead the path to a social insurance system. This compensation act had typical structures of an insurance system. Two years later the law of "old age pensions act" passed. It granted all needy citizens over 70 years a pension. 1911 also the national insurance law passed and health insurance as well as unemployment insurance made their way. Based on the "Beveridge-Reports" 1946 the "National Insurance Act", "National Health Service Act" and the "National Assistance Act" as well as the child allowance passed the law. These are still the basis for the British social system.[13]

2.2 Political background

The international comparison of the British social system is really interesting as Schmid states. It is a mixture of diverse kinds of welfare state systems.
- welfare state: universal conservative welfare state: insurance service dominate demand orientated services
- liberal welfare state: insurance services do not cover income
- social democratical social security system - all citizens are involved – and also for the significance of public production of welfare services

The British system can be called a liberal-collectivist system. The institution of market and family still play a great role and the security only gains relevance when those collapse. The fee financed insurance services provide only for the basic needs of the citizen. The amount of money which replaces the income is pretty low.
The British Beveridge system is based on the idea of citizenship. It means that each citizen has social rights. The three major rights are broad risk insurance, adequate insurance service and universality. Transferred to real life this means that every citizen in social needs has the right – no matter which job or salary the person earns – to get adequate welfare service.

---

[12] Mohr 2007
[13] Schmid 2002

Beveridge's concept is based on three assumptions:
the salary earned from working is the major source of income
the politico-economic goal of full employment is reached
full employment means "male full employment"

Obviously the last aspect causes controversial opinions. The welfare system of
Beveridge still relys on the traditional role of the women to be at home caring about
the household. But due to economical and society developments these things have
changed. This is also visible on the fact that dole money gained so much importance
compared to other social welfare services. So it should be adapted due to past and
current developments.[14]

2.3 Individual insurance

Accordig to Schmid the British welfare system is divided into three pillars. Firstly
there is the general social insurance the "national insurance". It covers the pension,
unemployment- and accident insurance as well as illness- and maternity allowance.
There are also other forms of social minimum collateral and also the National Health
Service (NHS). The NHS is subordinated from the Department of Social Security.
All employed citizens whose income is over the contribution assessment ceiling pay
contributions which match their income and the half of it is payed by the employer.
Social security insurance and the NHS are basically tax financed.

2.3.1 Pension

The pension insurance grants flat basic pension. To get the full pension citizens have
to pay 90 % of their working live into the pension fund. The basic pension one only
gets when he/she is under the 90 % and it is pretty low indeed, it is about the salary
of an industry worker. There are also widow payments but those depend on age and
amount of children. Private pension insurances gain importance for they can replace
the general pension insurance. Especially the conservative party supports privatized
pension insurances to relieve the public insurances.

2.3.2 Health care

The payment of sickness benefits is covered by the public welfare. When there is the
inability to work the insurance pays the salary for a maximum of half a year. The
services of the NHS – which are freely accessible for every citizen of the UK – are
pretty broad and include ambulant and stationary services as well as services of
specialized physicians. The ambulant services are mainly carried out by general
practitioners. The stationary services are mainly carried out by public hospitals. Due
to the health care reform in 1990 the stationary care is more open for private bidder.
Co-payments exist in the areas of dental care and drugs. But groups of people with
low salaries are excluded form co-payments. Private insurance companies are can

---

[14] Schmid 2002

only be found in the areas of co-payment. But since the abolishment tax relief's the amount of people who are privately insured stagnated.[15]

2.3.3 Family

The British welfare system includes maternity allowance and child allowance. Based on income and fee the maternity allowance gets paid. Women working since at least six month at the same workplace get a special allowance of 90 % of the current income in the first six weeks. For the next 12 weeks they get another flat rate.
No matter of the salary parents get a flat rate, tax financed child allowance until their child is 16 years old. For single parent the amount is higher.[16]

2.3.4 Accident insurance

The accident insurance is part of the general social insurance system. The insurance includes services in case of injuries, illness or death as a result of working accident. In case of disability the people get a pension.[17]

2.3.5 Unemployment

In GB there is the Jobseeker's Allowance (JSA) for unemployed citizen. This system combines contribution-based JSA and also income-based JSA which starts after 182 days of being unemployed. Everybody is allowed to get JSA who is not arbitrary without work or does not work than 16 or more hours per week. These job seekers have to show up in the jobcentres regularly and they also have to take jobs which are under their past income level.
Another central element of politicians is the New Labour Welfare-to-Work-Program "New Deal". It is for young people, long-term unemployed people, single parents and over 50 years old people. These people get specialized treatment and continuing education.[18]

3 To put in a nutshell

According to Mohr is Germany a typical coordinated market economy whereas GB is a liberal market economy. GB has one of the leastt deregulated markets of all OECD countries (2004). The educational system is not very job orientated unlike it is in Germany. The British system is described as "low skill equilibrium". The Economy is based on low qualified work with low productivity. "High-skill/high-wage" economy is Germany called. The educational standards are pretty high and income is relatively alike for every worker.
The welfare systems of Germany and the GB differ a lot. The German system is conservative and very much income depended which is likely to keep the current life

---

[15] Schmid 2002
[16] Schmid 2002
[17] Schmid 2002
[18] Schmid 2002

status. The "Unemployment Welfare Regime" of GB is liberal and it focuses rather on proverty proved minimum collateral. The GB system only provides the minimum of financial compensation for the unemployed. In Germany the minimum collateral is higher but a lot of unemployed people do not have the demand to claim for services because the requirements are pretty high. The system forces a division of "insider" and "outsider".[19]

4 Evaluation of welfare states

The comparison of welfare states can show some progress. From the methodical point of view there are better analysis, higher case numbers, reliable data and the statistical evaluation tools improve steadily.
There are also new concepts which connect the three areas of politics, policy and polity like Esping-Andersens did. And they also tried to put together the historical-sociological background.
Another topic is that not the quality of data rises but rather the quantity.
The focus on monetary data – easily available through OECD statistics – lead to the conclusion that this might be the only factor that really counts. But still it is difficult to look at the three areas of welfare state, private households and market.
Systematically analysis of social security and instruments and the interests of the involved parties are not high enough appreciated. The most studies focus on public institutions and politics and stay within the borders of a "social insurance state". But in this case the welfare pluralism and the third sector of welfare production is excluded. The effect on the typical structure of the welfare state and the employment systems get neglected. The way it is in Germany that most parts of the social and health care system is financed by the government and the welfare association with one Mio. employees provide 2/3 of the services. Schmid even shows solutions how comparison of welfare states can be improved. For the problem of too high qualification he insists to do efficiency and impact analysis as well as evaluate the interests of the people involved.
To keep from only focussing on the social security state Schmid's solution is to also involve welfare pluralism and welfare associations to widen the perspective.[20]

---

[19] Mohr 2007
[20] Schmid 2002

References

Braasch P., Das Gesundheitswesen in Deutschland: Struktur- Leistungen- Weiterentwicklung. 4th edit. 2007. Deutscher Ärzte Verlag

Schmid J., Wohlfahrtsstaaten im Vergleich. 2nd edit. 2002. Leske + Budrich UTB

Mohr K., Soziale Exklusion im Wohlfahrtsstaat: Arbeitslosensicherung und Sozialhilfe in Großbritannien und Deutschland. Verlag für Sozialwissenschaften